GetWaistedNOW: Little Book of Codes to Unlock Your Waistline

I0408456

Cynthia Marie Henderson

Dedication

"GetWaistedNOW: Little Book of Codes to Unlock Your Waistline" is dedicated to Angela Stewart (Cookie), Gwen Mickerson (Yung), Seandre' Hawkins (She-She), Tameka Young (Carmicita), Karey Satterwhite-Alexander (Rea), Tiffany, O'Mari, and O'Maya Willis (my family), and Ardella D. Fowler (Mickie aka my 9 to 5 mom and god-mother). I especially love, honor, and appreciate each of you for your kind words of encouragement, support, and gentle push as I walk INTO my divine purpose to help women re-invent and supersize their lives through sound health and wellness.

Namaste.

Preface

GetWaistedNow: Little Book of Codes to Unlock Your Waistline" came about in bite-size pieces over the last 5 years. After searching for ways to get well naturally, lose weight, and increase my vitality, I stumbled upon bits of information on the World Wide Web--a tip here, an adjustment there. At the time, I just couldn't find the information I desired all in one place, at least in an easy to read and direct to the point format. And when I did, I simply didn't have the time or energy to decipher through a 300 page book on how to do x, y, and z.

I am someone who has fought through yo-yo everything--weight gain, weight loss, eat well, eat badly—now realizing I have to make peace with food and intuitively trust the process. In my journey, I discovered one pivotal point-I had to get well, in order to get well. Getting well required me to implement small changes (mind, body, spirit) daily--the compound effect operating at its best. A "LITTLE" book of codes was written for the overwhelmed single mom, the super busy executive female who has lost focus on her health, or the female college student who has taken on a full class load, works full-time, and is on her way to gaining the "freshman 20". You see, I know all too well what it feels like to have life happen and lose myself. I was laid off from corporate America, unemployable because I was overqualified, then anxiety kicks in, insomnia kicks in, and slowly the weight creeps back. I thought I had it under control, but then my disabled sister goes blind right before my eyes and I felt guilty, as if it were my fault. Then my god-mother becomes gravely ill, later has a stroke, and a host of health concerns pop up. I became completely numb at the thought of possibly losing her and for the 5 months following her stroke, I visited with her in the hospital and rehabilitation center. I lost myself and found all the weight and bad habits I had previously lost too. Then one day it happened: I gazed in the mirror and didn't recognize myself. There's an old saying that goes "shit or get off the pot". Well, I didn't like what I saw and just like a few years earlier, I had lost the weight and totally transformed, I knew I could do it again! Getting off the pot was not an option for me. So my journey now continues with a new gym, a new personal trainer, a new set of awareness', and a positive mindset that re-invention is an awesome thing!

Use the "LITTLE" book of codes as stepping stones, small advancements that would ultimately lead to discovering your waistline again.

Cheers to your health, wellness, and getting WaistedNOW!

GetWaistedNOW: Little Book of Codes to Unlock Your Waistline Table of Contents

Why GetWaistedNow?

Family reunion, little black dress event, or boyfriend's annual company cookout--whatever the event, you can GetWaistedNOW! An event isn't really needed; all you need is the desire to make a quick change just to boost confidence and jumpstart your health goals.

Belly fat, that live fat, is one of the hardest fats to get rid of if you don't know what to do. GetWaistedNOW tackles numerous codes I discovered that actually work to help trim my waistline. Fat is stubborn and in case you didn't know, fat can shrink, but it never goes completely away. That's why when someone trims down, then re-gains, the fat seems to come back worse the next go-round. Researchers have discovered that fat cells can grow as much as 10 times their normal size. On some of us, that could be...well...let's just say–not the look we would like to achieve. Let's work toward shrinking them for good.

Remember this key thing about fat:

Fat cells can increase at any time, if you consistently consume more than your body burns off. So, if/when fat cells reach their **maximum size**, it looks to other fat cells to help it increase in **number**, which explains how some people experience rapid weight gain.

Code 1 - Drink Your Water

Drink water, drink your water, and drink water. Occasionally, I have to remind myself to get in enough water as well. Let's face it, our bodies are at least half water and it's a part of every single organ and cell. Without adequate water, our kidney and liver functions would come to a crawl and our bodies would not be able to rid themselves of waste in a proper manner. Water carries nutrients and oxygen to our cells, regulates our body temperature, keeps our skin looking refreshed, provides a feeling of fullness (which can prevent overeating), and helps to rid our body of excess waste. And although water is present in foods and beverages, there is nothing like pure water for proper organ and cell functioning. Have some water-it's calorie-free, gluten-free, cholesterol-free but more importantly, it's super refreshing. Take your water intake from good to great by drinking alkaline water. And if you have problems consuming enough water, try drinking it using a straw.

Code 1a - Get Jiggy With Your Water

Water may be calorie-free, gluten-free, cholesterol-free and super refreshing but in order to GetWaistedNOW, check out a few jiggy ideas to try with water:

Apple Cider Vinegar is a bit harsh to the taste buds, but the benefits can be phenomenal if you add just one tablespoon a day to a cup of pure warm water, preferably upon rising. It can promote healthy blood sugar levels, improve nutrient absorption, and aid in weight loss to name a few benefits. Be certain to get Apple Cider Vinegar with the **MOTHER**. In French, vinegar means "sour wine". Organic, unfiltered, Apple Cider Vinegar also contains "mother" which are strands of proteins, enzymes, and friendly bacteria that gives the vinegar a cloudy, cobweb-like appearance. If you can't tolerate the taste alone, add the juice of ½ fresh lemon.

If you really want to get jiggy with your water, try **Wheatgrass**. According to the Hippocrates Health Institute, Wheatgrass juice is nature's finest medicine. A mere 2 oz. has the nutritional equivalent of five pounds of the best raw organic vegetables. It has twice the amount of Vitamin A as carrots, is higher in Vitamin C than oranges, and contains the full spectrum of B vitamins. It's also a complete source of protein that supplies all of your amino acids. It's a detoxifier of the liver and the blood. It cleanses the body from head-to-toe of any heavy metals, pollutants, and other toxins that may be stored in the body's tissues or organs. Raw wheatgrass juiced is the best for you, but if you can't get a hold of freshly squeezed juice, opt for wheatgrass powder. Mix 1 tablespoon in 2 oz. of water twice a day. Do not exceed 4 oz. in a day.

Then, there is nature's best kept secret-**Chaga**. Chaga is a type of Siberian Mushroom. It's been used for thousands of years by various cultures and is very popular in Asian medicine. Chaga has key chemical compounds with a huge range of therapeutic benefits to include anti-tumor, anti-inflammatory, anti-microbial, anti-viral, anti-oxidant, and anti-cancer. The bottom line is that this powerhouse just may change the course of one's entire health! Chaga can be found in the form of a capsule. Drink it as a tea by opening up the capsule and emptying the contents into 4 oz. of pure warm water. This allows for quicker absorption by the body. Do not exceed the dosage amount noted by its' manufacturer.

These jiggy ideas are **IN ADDITION TO** drinking pure water daily.

Code 1b - Infused Water

Infused water is all the rage in the weight loss community. Why? Simply because it helps make our pure water slightly tasteful and helps to diminish belly bloat. Let's face it, some of the other codes may take more than a day or two before you notice a difference; but, infused water is bound to show up by way of less puffiness or bloat within 24 hours of drinking it. There are zillions of combinations on how to make infused water. My favorite is using 1 organic lemon, 1 organic cucumber, a few mint leaves, and 1 navel orange. Simply slice it all up, put the slices in the bottom of a pitcher, and add 2 cups of ice. Then, fill the pitcher up with pure water. Place the pitcher in the fridge for 2 hours or, better yet, overnight. Enjoy the contents throughout the following day. Hold off on the lemon until the next morning if you decide to let your infusion marinate overnight. The lemon tends to become extremely bitter the longer it sits.

Code 2 - Dry Brushing

Have you ever wondered what the funny looking brush or glove found in the personal care aisle was for? It's certainly not for brushing your hair. How about brushing your body? Yes, you can brush your body to health! Your largest organ, your skin, needs care and attention too! It's the first organ to show visible signs when it's being neglected. So give your skin a little T.L.C. daily. Why dry brush daily? It increases circulation to the skin helping to break down stored toxins in the body's fat. It helps shed dead skin cells and encourages new cell renewal. It also rejuvenates the nervous system by stimulating nerve endings in the skin. Dry brushing can even help with muscle tone and can give you more even fat deposits according to the source www.mindbodygreen.com

Tip: Dry brush every morning. Start on dry skin before bathing. Work brush or glove in a circular, upward motion. Begin at your ankles and move upward towards your heart. Hop in the shower and rinse away the dead skin cells. Follow your refreshing shower with a moisturizer such as coconut oil or emu oil.

Code 3 - Supp Your Gut

Sometimes our guts leak. Toxins and undigested food escape from the digestive system and travel throughout the body via the bloodstream. As a result, our body does not absorb the nutrients it needs to function properly. When this happens, we may experience bloat, flatulence or even worse, weight gain. And no matter the amount of good foods we eat plus those 2 hours in the gym, we simply don't see any changes on the scale or in our clothes. The bottom line is: until we heal our gut, we won't lose our butt! A simple fix to GetWaistedNOW and to help heal the gut–Probiotics! Sure, you can eat foods containing probiotics like raw dandelion greens, raw onions, or raw asparagus, yogurt, sauerkraut, miso soup or pickles, but who wants to limit their diets to eating that every day? Not to mention the amount you would need to eat in order to make a significant difference in your gut restoration is difficult to rationalize. Therefore, the best probiotics to take are in the form of supplements. For improved digestive health, definitely add those foods to your diet; but, also add a quality probiotic supplement to your daily regime too. The verdict is out on the amount needed. Some research suggests taking a minimum of 25 billion CFU's (Colony Forming Units) as this amount is essential to restoring the good bacteria and healing the gut. Remember to nourish your system with those real foods noted above so that the probiotics can balance the ratio of beneficial bacteria to bad bacteria in your gut.

Code 4 - Cleanse/Detox

Just like warning indicators flash on our cars' dashboard when gas is low, tire pressure is deflating, or the engine is running hot, our bodies give us signals that we need to pause and check something out. Infrequent bowel movements, skin rashes or flare ups like eczema, frequent colds, bloat, brain-fog, constant headaches, or steady weight gain-has any of these conditions 'copped a squat' in your body's home? Well, these might be sure-fire symptoms that a cleanse/detox regimen may be needed.

Cleanses and detoxes are actually one and the same. The terms are used interchangeably but they both have the same goal associated with it: rid the body of toxins. And once the body rids itself of toxins, it begins to heal and start functioning more at optimum levels–inflammation subsides, skin begins to clear and even glow, hair becomes shinier, and nails become stronger just to name a few benefits. Juicing and plant-based eating are primary ways to cleanse/detox allowing the digestive system to rest. In return, the body purges built up toxic waste via the evacuation channels. Although our bodies are designed to cleanse themselves on their own; with the overconsumption of alcohol, tobacco, and processed foods, air pollution, and the overuse of medication and supplements, these factors make it harder to do so.

Don't think long-term when doing a cleanse/detox regimen. Typically, they should be completed in a pre-set number of days-anywhere from 1 to 21 days-any longer than that can be dangerous. Severely restricting food makes it hard to get the proper nutrients our body needs. Decreased energy, drop in blood sugar levels, as well as, electrolyte imbalances can occur from long-term cleanse/detox regimens. The biggest danger is its ability to bring our metabolism to a screeching halt; thus making it harder to lose weight. So think short-term, as it's a way for the body to begin the healing process naturally.

Code 5 - Yes, Go Meatless

Give it a break once in a while--the meat! Since 2003, there's been a Meatless Monday campaign sweeping the globe. It's based on the premise that skipping meat at least 1 day a week is good for healthier living and better for the planet. Who doesn't want to reduce their carbon footprint and save freshwater sources?

Diabetes, heart disease, some forms of cancers, and obesity are just some of the diseases that can be eliminated if we reduce our meat consumption according to Meatless Monday proponents. Going meatless also encourages more plant-based eating. You'll get more folate, fiber, zinc, iron and magnesium when consuming more vegetables, beans or peas according to Mitchell DC, Lawrence FR, Hartman TJ, Curran JM (2009) "Consumption of Dry Beans, Peas, Lentils Could Improve Diet Quality in the U.S. Population." Journal of the American Dietetic Association 109(5):909-13.

Diets with a higher intake of plant-based proteins instead of meats can result in fewer deaths due to cardiovascular issues. So eat your fruits, vegetables (cooked and raw), grains such as quinoa and lentils, and raw nuts to become healthier and GetWaistedNOW!

If going meatless for one entire day seems daunting, try going meatless at 1 main meal a few times a week. Once you get use to enjoying plant-based eating, (and you will) trying going meatless at two meals a day a few times a week. Finally, once you are totally comfortable with eating meatless, go meatless the entire day the next Monday in honor of Meatless Monday!

I thought I would lose my mind if I didn't have chicken at every meal but then I discovered Portobello mushrooms, tempeh, black beans, and falafel (chickpeas). Once you go meatless and incorporate more plant-based eating, be certain to add healthy fats such as avocado, raw cashews, or pumpkin seeds in moderation. These healthy fats help your body assimilate the green vegetables easily.

One of my favorite meatless snacks is Ezekiel Bread (toasted) with almond butter and a sliced ripe banana on top. It's not only delicious, it's filling, it's healthy and it has the right balance to help fuel my workout or simply hold me over until my next meal. For a pdf of meatless recipes provided by the Meatless Monday campaign go to: http://bit.ly/mmcomfort2

Code 6 - Go Raw, Go Green (or Go Home)

Yuck! Ewww! Umph! I know that's what comes to mind when you think about eating raw foods. Well, the Raw Food Revolution is here to stay! It's trending now! You'll go raw, go green, or go home! Hopefully, you'll go raw and watch how you GetWaistedNOW by adding more raw foods into your life! Eating a green salad is just the beginning of eating raw. A real raw-food-diet consists of eating more seasonal and unprocessed foods in order to get a variety of nutrients that your body calls for without the added chemicals, fertilizers, pesticides, and food additives. The benefits of eating raw include less inflammation, improved digestion, more fiber, more energy, improved heart health, and weight loss to name a few. In other words eating raw may be healing.

The potential hydrogen (a.k.a pH) is something that determines whether a food or drink is acidic or alkaline. Raw foods alkalize the pH level in our bodies. Disease cannot live in an alkaline environment. This simply means overly-cooked foods are likely to create an acidic environment in the body allowing our health to slowly deteriorate; while raw foods help to create an alkaline environment helping our body to be free of disease.

I'm not suggesting you go 100% raw. The transition from red meat, processed foods, and refined sugars to eating 100% or perhaps even 50% raw could put anyone in an uproar; so, slowly adding raw fruits and vegetables daily, in combination with, lightly cooked, steamed foods, as well as green smoothies are ideal. By the way, food is considered raw if it's prepared at 118 degrees Fahrenheit or below.

Some staples in your raw food diet would include: leafy greens such as kale, spinach, or chard. Then there's' broccoli, cabbage, asparagus, celery, cilantro, cucumbers, melons, apple, mango, bananas, avocados, wild rice, quinoa, almonds, pine nuts, chia seeds, flax seeds, hemp seeds, extra virgin olive oil, flaxseed oil, stevia, herbal teas, alkaline water, cayenne pepper, garlic, ginger, oregano, turmeric, Himalayan salt, dark chocolate with 70% or higher cacao content, bee pollen, royal jelly, spirulina, chlorophyll. The best part of these staples is that some of them can be thrown in the mix when you blend a green smoothie taking it from good and making it great!

I absolutely love www.incrediblesmoothies.com website. You can find a plethora of information on how to correctly build a delicious green smoothie. This has been my favorite go-to reference website for years. The recipes are easy to follow and turn out delicious.

Don't make eating raw hard. It can be a simple as snacking on sliced bell peppers, especially red peppers, with cilantro hummus as a dip. Talk about yummy!

When eating raw, be sure to note the Dirty Dozen/Clean Fifteen lists of fruits and vegetables-to eat conventionally or purchase organically-found at www.ewg.org When all else fails, buy from your local farmers.

Code 7 - Walk It Out

As boring as a brisk walk may be, it's vital in order to **GetWaistedNOW**. Walking has so many benefits which include toning your calves, quads and hamstrings, while lifting your glutes. Posture yourself upright, contract your abdominal muscles while walking, and you'll tone up those abs and shrink your waistline. Walking also strengthens your heart muscle. Enjoy it outside regularly and you will even boost your Vitamin D levels-something many people in the United States are deficient in. In case you didn't know, a Vitamin D deficiency can result in a dramatic loss of energy, stunt weight loss efforts, and create muscle weakness. On your annual visit to your primary care doctor, be certain to ask them to check your Vitamin D levels.

I can recall one year where my Vitamin D levels were fewer than 12-along with my Iron levels reading at 7. My doctor looked at me with a serious face and asked how in the world I was still walking around. I later found out that between 30 to 50 mL is considered a good Vitamin D range for healthy people, while anything less than 12 is considered deficient. Needless to say, my doctor flooded me with high dosages of prescribed Vitamin D therapy and Iron. I never realized that feeling sluggish was not normal. I had been run-down for so long that I thought that was how I naturally felt.

Finally, walking can boost your mood, warding off depression, anxiety, and stress. Now, if those aren't awesome reasons to walk it out...

MY DELICIOUS
DISCOVERIES

Arugula Detox Salad

2 Handfuls of Organic Arugula
English Cucumber (sliced)
½ Avocado (cubed)
½ Cup of Radish (thinly sliced)
Handful of Cilantro
1 Tbsp. Flaxseed

Dressing

2 Tbsps. Extra Virgin Olive Oil
1 Tbsp. Braggs Apple Cider Vinegar
½ Lemon (squeeze)

OR

My personal favorite:
Newman's Own Organics Olive Oil & Vinegar

Many studies suggest that Arugula may decrease the risk of obesity, diabetes, heart disease and overall mortality while promoting a healthy complexion, increased energy, and overall lower weight. *Arugula contains a high amount of Vitamin K, if you are taking blood-thinners, please check with your personal physician before consuming.

Cabbage Hemp Detox Salad

Red Cabbage (shredded)
½ Avocado
¼ Organic Red Pepper
¼ Organic Yellow Pepper
Handful of Cilantro

Dressing

2 Tbsps. Extra Virgin Olive Oil
1 Tbsp. Braggs Apple Cider Vinegar
½ Lemon (squeeze)

OR

My personal favorite:
Newman's Own Organics Olive Oil Vinegar

Cabbage is rich in Fiber, Vitamin C, Iodine and Sulphur. Its' health benefits range from treating constipation, skin disorders like eczema, headaches, and bleeding gums to alleviating ulcers, promoting sound eye health, and boosting mental clarity. It's also a popular vegetable to eat when trying to lose weight since it's filling and very low in calories.

Pad Thai

1 Zucchini (spiraled thick)
1 Large Carrot (spiraled thick) or Bag of Shredded Carrots
Organic Green Onions (finely chopped)
½ Organic Red Pepper (sliced thinly)
Mung Bean Sprouts

Thoroughly wash all vegetables. Use a spiraler to spiral the zucchini and carrot. Thinly chop the green onions and slice the red pepper. Be sure to clean the seeds from the inside of the pepper. Combine all ingredients in a small bowl.

Sauce*

4 Tbsp. of Almond Butter
Pc of Ginger
1 Tbsp. Braggs Amino
1 Clove of Garlic (peeled)
1 Tbsp. Agave
1 Tsp. of Cayenne Pepper
(2 Tbsps. Thinly Copped Cashews SET ASIDE FOR GARNISH)

Blend all sauce ingredients until smooth. If a blender is not available, simple use a fork to wisk ingredients. Immediately spoon 2-3 tbsps. onto combined ingredients and Enjoy! This is, by far, one of my favorite recipes.

Hummin' Hummus

1 Can of Garbanzo Beans
½ Tbsp. Cumin
½ Tsp. Tahini
1 Garlic Clove (minced)
1 Tbsp. flaxseeds
¼ Lemon (squeeze)

Preserve ¼ cup of liquid from Garbanzo Beans. Blend all ingredients and slowly add preserved liquid to blender if mixture becomes too thick. Once blended to desired consistency, spoon into a bowl, and cover with a lid. Refrigerate for 2 hours.

My Beets Don't Kale My Vibe

4-5 Golden Beets
Organic Curly Kale Leaves
Extra Virgin Olive Oil
¼ Lemon (squeezed)

(Seasonings)
Pepper
Garlic & Leek Seasonings
Thyme

Wash golden beets and curly kale thoroughly. Slice them into the size of wedges. Season them with pepper, garlic & leek seasoning, and thyme. Layer your beets on a cookie sheet. Drizzle extra virgin olive oil over beets and coat thoroughly. Bake beets on 325 degrees until tender. While they are baking pat dry curly kale. Stir fry curly kale in extra virgin olive oil. Layer kale and beets in a bowl and enjoy!

The Smoothie is King

Apple Detox Smoothie

Large Handful of Dandelion Greens
½ Lemon (squeezed)
1 Large Green Apple
1 Banana (spotted)
1-2 Tbsps. of Flaxseed
6 oz. of Spring Water

Blend all ingredients with a few ice cubes. Drink immediately!

Everything but the kitchen Sink Smoothie

Handful of Organic Baby Spinach & Organic Baby Kale
English Cucumber (sliced)
¼ Avocado
2 Tbsps. of Flaxseeds
2 Large Navel Oranges
½ Cup of Blueberries or Mixed Berries (frozen)
½ Lemon (squeeze)
Small Handful of Cilantro
5-6 Organic Mint Leaves
8 oz. of Spring Water

Blend all ingredients with a few ice cubes. Drink immediately!

The Smoothie is King

Paradise Smoothie

Handful of Organic Baby Kale
1 Cup of Fresh Pineapple
¼ Avocado
½ Cup of Cherries
½ Lemon (squeeze)
5-6 Organic Mint Leaves
8 oz. of Spring Water

Blend all ingredients with a few ice cubes. Drink immediately!

Basic Smoothie

Handful of Organic Baby Spinach
English Cucumber
1 Large Navel Orange
1/2 Banana (spotted)
¼ Cup of Cashews
½ Lemon (squeeze)
8 oz. of Spring Water

Blend all ingredients with a few ice cubes. Drink immediately!

NOTES

[   ] *I absolutely love the* _____
     and wouldn't change a thing.
[   ] *I loved this but need to modify it a little bit.*
[   ] *I didn't enjoy this at all.*

Modifications:

_____

_____
_____
_____
_____
_____
_____
_____
_____
_____
_____
_____
_____
_____
_____
_____
_____
_____
_____
_____
_____
_____
_____
_____
_____
_____
_____
_____

NOTES

[   ] *I absolutely love the* _____
     and wouldn't change a thing.
[   ] *I loved this but need to modify it a little bit.*
[   ] *I didn't enjoy this at all.*

Modifications:

_____

_____
_____
_____
_____
_____
_____
_____
_____
_____
_____
_____
_____
_____
_____
_____
_____
_____
_____
_____
_____
_____
_____

Contraindications

WHOLElisticallySpeaking, LLC does not claim to diagnose, prescribe, treat, or cure any disease or illness. Individual results from "**GetWaistedNOW: Little Book of Codes to Unlock Your Waistline**" may vary. No individual results should be seen as typical.

Those who have any health issues, who are pregnant or nursing, diabetic, have Celiac Disease, or have sensitivities to Wheatgrass, should consult with their personal physician.

If you have infrequent bowel movements, Sarcoidosis, Heart Disease, Kidney Stones or Kidney Disease, consult with your personal physician before consuming apple cider vinegar.

And lastly, if you are on blood-thinning medication, avoiding dark green leafy vegetables may be key, as the Vitamin K may interfere with the effectiveness of your medication. Consult with your personal physician before consuming dark green leafy vegetables.

Resource Guide

Books	
Reference Book	**Author**
The Encyclopedia of Healing Foods *"A comprehensive guide from A to Z on nutritional benefits and medicinal properties of food w/food prescriptions form common ailments."*	Michael Murray, N.D.
Fast Food, Good Food *"150 quick and easy ways to put healthy, delicious foods on the table."*	Andrew Weil, M.D.
Eat to Live *"Nutrient rich program for fast and sustained weight loss Health=nutrients/calories" Revised 2011*	Dr. Joel Fuhrman, MD
Website	
www.mindbodygreen.com *"Website with a mission to help revitalize the way people eat, move, and live."*	
www.incredibalesmoothies.com *"The Green Smoothie lifestyle with recipes and tips on weight loss and health".*	
www.livestrong.com *"Diet nutrition and fitness tips for a healthier lifestyle."*	
YouTube	
Fitlifetv	
Food Matters	
Kris Carr	
Fullyrawkristina	
Healers/Coaches/Motivators	
Reference Book	**Author**
Who Moved My Cheese *"A funny short story on how to deal with change in your life."*	Spencer Johnson, MD
Grow Younger, Live Longer *"Practical step by step program designed to show how it is essential to renew all dimensions of the self-the body, mind, and spirit in order to feel and look younger."*	Deepak Chopra
No Matter What *"Nine steps to living the life you want."*	Lisa Nichols
How to Heal with Color – Balance Your Chakras *"Rejuvenate your health; learn colors for common ailments."*	Ted Andrews

Find Me On Social Media

Facebook: @WHOLElisticllySpeaking

Twitter: cmarieunitea

Instagram: c_m_henderson

Email: wholelisticallyspeaking@yahoo.com